SWEET AND BITTER FOOL

A priest's journey through manic depression

D1797946

PHILIP CLEMENTS

"One million people commit suicide every year"
World Health Organisation

Published by:
Chipmukapublishing
PO Box 6872
Brentwood
Essex
CM13 1ZT
United Kingdom

www.chipmunkapublishing.com

Dedicated to my very patient and supportive family and friends. Christmas 2003.

The poems I have written and interspersed between some of the chapters may help to throw light on some of my feelings and experiences. P.C.C.

A word of thanks.

My grateful thanks to those who have stood by me and who tried to understand.
Special thanks to my mother and other members of the family.

Amongst my friends, my thanks to those at Lancing and in my former parishes of Ninfield and Hooe. In addition my gratitude to the late Father Dennis Rankin, Daff and Dr. Kemm. Thank-you too for those doctors and nurses who were a real help, also my analyst. A big thank you too to all who prayed and willed me to be well again finally, Deo Gratias on bad days and on good.

Philip Clements.

SYNOPSIS

This book is the description of an Anglican priest's experience of manic depression.

In it he relates what may have been early signs of obsession and depression when he was a teenager. The author describes events leading up to his first breakdown as a student at university preparing for ordination. His career continues largely unabated until a second depressive episode soon after starting an important appointment. When he was admitted to hospital, it was as if all his hopes and aspirations had ended. He later resumed his ministry and after nine years he moved to take charge of two rural parishes. Hardly had he started that another major episode occurred. In a suicidal state he went to hospital again, and then for a longer period, to a private hospital.

Nothing availed and the author is critical of some of the treatment received.

Nothing seemed to succeed until more drastic treatment was attempted when back at home. Later and after about thirty years following his first breakdown, the G.P. in his parish diagnosed manic depression and prescribed lithium. Since then the author fulfilled an active and lively ministry for nine years until he retired .

The book describes the depths of the illness and at the same time, a ministry which somehow survived successfully despite occasional interruptions.

The story continues in an active retirement with the illness largely controlled by lithium. The book relates the illness in all its awfulness, but it also testifies to its management once it is properly diagnosed. Manic depression is powerful but the sufferer need not be overwhelmed and can still live and achieve against all odds and expectations.

> 'Do thou for him stand:
> The sweet and bitter fool
> Will presently appear;
> The one in motley here,
> The other found out

there…'

> (Shakespeare-'King

Lear' Act 1,Scene 4)

About the Author.

Philip was born in 1938. As World Was 2 was ending
he moved with his family from Manchester to a Kentish
village near Dover. He was then nearly seven. He went
to the local primary school and later the Grammar
school in Dover. On leaving school he worked in a
library in Deal and Sandwich. After a year at a school
of librarianship, he became a children's librarian.
Feeling called to the Anglican Ministry, he studied at
King's College London, and at Theological College.
In 1965 he was ordained and became a Curate in South
Norwood. Then for twenty two years he was a School
Chaplain and teacher in Croydon, Staffordshire and
Sussex. In 1990 he became Vicar and Rector to two
rural parishes near Battle in East Sussex. He retired to
Kent in 1999 at the age of sixty. Here he o been active
in helping in parishes, in working for Christian unity,
and in writing and broadcasting. He has published four
books of poetry in limited editions.
'Poems of Youth.' 1987.

'Deal Pier.' 2001.

'The Plague of 2001.' 2002

'Words in you ear'. 2004

In much of his life he has suffered manic depressive episodes but has somehow come through.

……………………………………………………………….

.

POEMS.

Sleep and rising.1992.
Fence. 1988.
Alone. 1988.
And it was night. 1987.
Breakdown. 1982.

(from Deal pier and other poems. 2001.)

Doubt. 1957.
Vanity, vanity. 1957.

(from 'Poems of Youth'1987).

Me or not to be? 2001.
Gone before. 2000.
In solitary. 1995.

(from 'The plague of 2001 and other poems.2002). .

INTRODUCTION.

Many have written of their experience of acute depression. I simply add my own personal testimony to their's, a record which is also an account of aspects of my ministry as an Anglican priest and the effects of the illness on my work. Once when particularly ill, I was seeking counsel from another priest, the Vicar of the parish where I was living. It happened to be a 'good day', or as I would now call it a 'manic day'. He looked at me straight in the eyes, and said quite seriously,' A breakdown doesn't bring any glory to God.' I do not think the full impact of this has yet come home, and perhaps I misheard him, or so I hope. True, I am a Christian priest, but what has happened to me during my life, has been hideous, and it would seem to have born not of sin or inadequacy, but of chemicals doing unpredictable things in my otherwise sane mind, albeit triggered by different causes.

So with that bit of unkindness out of the way, I will describe what has happened to me, how it felt to be ill, and how I survived the worst and blackest onslaughts.

At this moment I rejoice that after fifty years of real illness, I am reasonably stable and well, as a result of medication and the understanding and prayers of many. I add to this my own will to survive and to pursue what I believe to be my vocation.

The tunnel we manic depressives go through is real, yet most of us, I believe, emerge into some degree of light. And surely it is here and not in the darkness that all are meant to be.   P.C.C.

CHAPTER   1

BEGINNINGS. 1955-1960.

Signs of an illness first came to me in the staff toilet of Deal Public Library where I was employed as a library assistant after leaving school. It was proving to be a difficult day. I was feeling what some would call 'moody'. I had experienced this before, as many people do, but I knew it wouldn't last and that I would soon resume my normal cheerful gregarious self. And so it proved, and I guess that no-one had taken any notice.

At home we had security, and though by no means affluent, we never lacked for the basics. There were the normal tensions between myself and my three younger brothers, and frustration and sometimes anger between my father and me, his teenage and precocious son. There was also much that was good: the village cricket team's matches for which I was often the scorer, trips to Dover, Deal and Folkestone for shopping and the beach, jolly birthdays with Mother's chocolate cake, and Christmases with the luxury, for those days, of poultry, Christmas pudding and home made mince pies ,sausage rolls and more cake. I was happy too at our village church where I had been head chorister and graduated to reading lessons at Evensong, and serving at Holy Communion. I also took part in concerts in the village hall and acted in the local Players. I had enjoyed my time at the village primary school and at my grammar school. How quickly these formative years passed.

One problem for me, emerging even then, was that I didn't always appreciate authority when it seemed loud and aggressive. My father had been in the army, and loved his sport. I was not sporty, but rather creative and imaginative. I was certainly not soldier material and had left the Combined Cadet Corps at school. Whenever I encountered a dominant male, we would clash sooner or later. I'm not blaming anyone, but even to this day, my inner strength flinches in the face of such a person, and yet at the same time I have found it difficult to express my own anger and frustration. Perhaps it is because I might have found such reaction incompatible with going to church and trying to be good. So in all this time I must have been accumulating a considerable amount of suppressed rage. And somehow it lacked outlets. So if depression is 'anger turned inwards', well then, there may be a starter here way back to my mid teens. But serious and clinical depression was a long way off, yet tiny clouds may have begun to herald the future storms.

After Deal I went for a year's study at the School of Librarianship, Loughborough College. Here I recall no depression. Homesickness, yes, but no 'black dog' as Winston Churchill described his black moods. Our teachers were good and they related to us well. I made some good friends, and I enjoyed acting in the College's production of 'Cymbeline'.

I passed my exams and returned to Deal, becoming the children's librarian. This too was a happy time. I felt I had achieved something for I was a qualified librarian. I began contributing to professional journals. I was awarded a Library Association prize, and traveled to the Midlands to receive it. I then made my first big move, living away from home in St.Albans where I worked in the College of Further Education. The college Librarian and his wife could not have been kinder, and I made good relationships with staff and students alike. I produced and acted in plays, and when I left, I donated a silver cup for drama. Again I do not recall being depressed. My faith was strong and I became a Server at the Abbey. How exciting it was walking along still empty streets to the silent early morning abbey, robing in the then unfamiliar robes and meeting the Celebrant, one of the cathedral dignitaries.

A little late even for that time, my sexuality was beginning to stir, yet I was not unduly concerned about its lateness, nor did I feel any serious guilt about its not developing as perhaps it should. I tried hard to find a girl friend, and took a female student to the cinema. Incidentally I now recall, when I was only six, having very strong feelings for a six year old girl on a Sunday school outing. She was a twin, and I couldn't be sure which of them I was with at any one time. When I was a teenager I fell for a girl at a holiday camp, but when it was over, so was the friendship. But now at about twenty, I began to feel particularly close to one or two of the male students who would come to supper from time to time. It was all very innocent and at the same time puzzling for someone who was ignorant about any kind of sexuality. There was also a strong friendship with someone a bit older than myself. We shared a room at our lodgings and he even came one weekend to meet my parents. I was devoted to him and didn't think to label what I felt, or have any sense of guilt. There wasn't anything to feel guilty about. The friendship was close but unphysical. Because of a degree of confusion, I adopted a largely celibate life style.

These were times without anger, but I imagine that the inner store of negativity was being added to, now perhaps being compounded by feelings of affection which I felt unable to express.

Why? No-one had told me about the different possibilities in relationships and degrees of affection. Television was just expanding and ignorance prevailed. My father was a 'Man's man' in the tough sense and was a kind of male stereotype. He was physically compact, sporty, enjoying matey talk with other men, speaking the language of soldiers and of the pub.

What was he to make of his eldest son, certainly not effeminate, but tidy and neatly dressed, reluctant to soil his hands, and speaking in a different way, acting in plays, singing in a church choir, working in libraries and writing poetry? My eyes must at times have registered disdain, and his mouth and eyes likewise. My mother always said,' He is proud of you', but he seemed unable to show it.

Then there was the Church. It didn't preach against particular forms of sexuality. It didn't feel the need to do so. Particular bits of the Bible that might have helped or hindered on this subject were not read or explained. Sex wasn't discussed generally and the popular media were 'unsullied'. My conscience was developing fast and was becoming dominant. It was the forum where all sources of 'good' influence converged. It became particularly troublesome if I thought I had caused anyone any hurt, or if I considered that I had been in the slightest bit dishonest. My conscience was in fact becoming tyrannical. I would sometimes grieve for days, until, almost bursting with despair, I would confess to my mother who was always my rock and consolation. She would dissipate the haunting thoughts, and again I would know peace, until conscience put me once more upon the rack. Of course so much of my anxiety was irrational. As for any kind of sex ,I had done nothing, which may have been a problem in itself.

So far then, it seems as if there were some seeds of a depressive illness, of which I was then blissfully unaware. The recognition is of course with hindsight. Repressed anger, repressed and uncertain sexuality and an overactive conscience and guilt formed a brew which was gently but certainly simmering. Yet I do not believe that these potent ingredients alone make for what developed later. They are probably in part the common lot of adolescence and emerging manhood.

There had to be something more, yet it was to take years or turmoil for the illness to be diagnosed and treated. It was not until 1990,over thirty years after the first signs and after three crippling breakdowns, that a G.P. who had an interest in psychiatric medicine, identified the problem and prescribed the right medication. Thank God that our paths coverged, but how different my life might have been if this treatment had begun years earlier. The miracle is that after this long period of manic depression, I had any life at all!

CHAPTER   2

GATHERING STORM. 1961-1963.

Illness is almost a contradiction of God. From an early age I was involved with religion and felt devout, and as a boy, I enjoyed being in the church choir, found religious education interesting and never questioned God's existence. In those early days when depression was beginning, I did not relate it to either religion or illness. They were separate worlds. I didn't see a doctor about feeling low and never mentioned it to a priest, or indeed to anyone. It was a small problem, a mild irritant. True there were mood swings, but these were not considered unusual, especially for a teenager.

My post school days as a library assistant, then as a student at the school of librarianship and finally as a Senior Library Assistant at the college in St.Albans, were largely happy and undisturbed by gloom. Maybe any unhappiness I might have known I have long since forgotten, but at this time there was no serious indication of what was lurking within my brain.

Emotionally I felt fairly happy though at times uneasy. After all, to have a girlfriend at this age was expected.

In my early twenties and at St.Albans, I decided to respond to a strong conviction of vocation to the Anglican Ministry. I was selected by the Church at a conference at St.Albans, and in 1961 I went to King's College, London, to its Theological Faculty, and to reside for the first two years at an inter-faculty Hall of Residence on Clapham Common. I enjoyed it all, and was even elected to the Hall committee because of my qualifications as a librarian. So I became Librarian of Halliday Hall and presided over a musty collection of drab looking books in a somewhat dingy and dark room.

My undoing or trigger was to stand for election as Hall Secretary or President as it was changed to. I was ambitious. I could not fail. I must be elected. I even had to learn a joke to relate at the hustings, as it was expected. But I had also heard that my rival for the post and a group of his friends had recently been a bit 'yobbish' at a Fair on the Common. I used this knowledge in my speech, accusing the other candidate of loutish behaviour. The vote was taken and I was elected by a large majority. I was elated but only temporarily. I was now top student, President Elect of a University Hall.

The next day at breakfast in college which followed the mid-week Communion, the Dean congratulated me. I felt awful. Grey fog seemed to dog every step. All joy disappeared. My appetite fled. There was darkness without limit. I couldn't face the defeated candidate. I even felt as if I had 'killed' him. I went to his room to apologize and to one or two of his group of friends. They didn't think much of me, but accepted what had happened with good grace.

The guilt was all pervading. At about that time my mother and one of my brothers   visited me at the Hall and we went to the Science Museum. It was a dark November day, perfectly reflected by my mood. I was even more distressed when their visit ended. I stopped going to lectures. I didn't want to go out at all. Close friends visited me in my room, but this was of little consolation. In the pit of my stomach was a dead weight. The tension in and around my head was relentless.

In was early in the morning of December the 8th, the Feast of the Conception of the Blessed Virgin Mary, and I was with friends at a mass at a convent across the Common. I began to lose consciousness and fell to the floor. I was brought round and taken back to Hall. I suppose my mind could take no further anxiety and guilt. I saw the Dean who arranged for me to see a doctor, a psychiatrist I think. He prescribed anti-depressants and a period of rest at home. The Christmas holidays were very near. The Hall Matron and her deputy could not have been kinder, allowing me to weep which I did easily and frequently, and wanting to give comfort. I was desolate, the future looked uncertain, and the tablets would take time.

So I went home, believing that a time with my family and a change of scenery would help. I was seen off at Victoria Station by friends and met at the other end by my mother. But Christmas is a bad time for depressives. I remember accompanying my father shopping in Dover and one of his friends greeting us cheerily. Every cheerful face added to my unhappiness. The town was decorated, everything was festive and people looked happy. Christ was being born again, and I just wanted to die. I envied my great aunts for being old. I was also perplexed about my feelings. I was on unfamiliar territory and the future was a blank wall.

Yet I fought. I went for walks and drove myself hard on cycle rides. I tried to employ my mind which by now was not only full of guilt, but becoming increasingly apprehensive about going back to college and becoming President.

I don't remember Christmas itself. I am sure that Mother, ever brave, tried her best for everyone's sakes. I couldn't have had a better mother throughout. My father was also supportive but I don't think he understood, yet he did assure me that I would always have a home. Of course the condition is such that the more support and sympathy are given, the deeper the darkness seems, as if the mind will only feed on guilt and misery reluctant to be helped. On one level the support is of course important. I don't remember how my brothers reacted at this time. Maybe they didn't notice though Charles who was also at the university training in dentistry, would prove extremely helpful soon and again much later when another episode occurred.

Christmas passed. I remember little except my own gloom. The depressed are enclosed within themselves. As January approached, I became very distressed particularly the night before I was due to return to London. I wept as I packed. How could I face it? The answer was 'I couldn't', so I contacted the Hall Warden. He wouldn't accept my resignation as Hall President, but I knew I couldn't return for some time. So I was given a 'stay of execution'. I began to feel better.

A week or two later I returned to Hall and College and to being President. I bought a date a day calendar, and by just tearing a day off at a time, I felt I was making progress. I planned and gave small parties for the other students. I seemed to succeed in making the House a friendlier place. None of this was easy, but I knew that most of the students were sympathetic, so I managed. The depression lifted but the feelings of guilt went on. I was also on top of my studies again. Sitting next to the Warden at dinner was difficult because he was very shy with no small talk. I would make a list of topics, but would sometimes get completely through them before the soup course was finished! Only once did I succeed. His subject was Classics, and I asked him a classical question. He talked through all the courses and through coffee in another room until only the two of us were left.

So the earlier blackness had not impeded me for long. This was to be the pattern of things. Earlier I had been suicidal at times. Now I was enjoying life and responsibility.

Charles helped relieve the 'Warden at dinner' problem by meeting me every Friday evening when we would go to a West End theatre and meal. At weekends the Warden ate elsewhere. So my college days continued largely untroubled. In my penultimate year in London, I was given a place amongst a dozen other ordinands from all over the country, to go to the Holy Land, to study on an eight week course at the Anglican Theological College in Jerusalem. This was an exciting prospect, but sadly it was to be seriously marred by something which was to feed my mental condition, and overshadow much of my life for more than twenty five years. It would be an ingredient in two further episodes of my illness.

Chapter 3 follows after poems.

'DOUBT'

Eagles to the clouds sore and wheel

From the gnarled pines.
Emblems of faith, incongruous doubt, to steal
From strongest and most wooden mines.

Venomous arrows from the bow
Of sneering friends,
Pierce the mounting spirits, and the shadowed glow,
Tattered and vanquished, yields and bends.

Clean through the heart the needle cuts,
And ruddy strength
Seeps. As the former shot, the target drops, ruts
The sky: a thud; it falls at length.

Inanimate it flies, and yet
Does cease to fly.

Faith, with the blood gone! Complacent bet,
Has for a moment won to try.

Is this the end? The breeze in man,
Resisting, stirs.
Inanimation fails, and doubt's weakened span
Strengthens the eagle's rising spurs.

1957(from 'Poems of
Youth')

VANITY,VANITY.

Illustrious spirit in the depths

Of the nursery of feelings.

Spring out and fall

Upon the earth.

But this is done.

Hence the dearth

Amongst our kinsfolk.

Unfeeling hindrance showered

From the outer person

Of an inner soul.

Pomp and glory

Are imagined and

The result: a sorry

Misconception of our actions.

The abdication of an

Honest man is made,

And lies become the outward

Form of truth;

Or truth becomes a dressy

Veil, and decency

Becomes an outward vesture

For deceptive state within.

1957(from 'Poems of Youth').

CHAPTER 3

FROM HEAVEN TO HELL.
1963-1968.

What of my faith in times of acute depression?
Basically it remained, but prayer and churchgoing
badly lapsed during the worst times. Prayer suffered
because I had little to say except for passionate and
repeated pleas for help. I do recall in my first episode
repeating the words 'Lord help me, the son of your
handmaid', clearly seizing upon scriptural fragments
when my mind had virtually ceased to operate
rationally. In my own style I was mute. I was unable to
concentrate on reading but later when the depression
lifted, I was to derive inspiration and help from the
poetry of a very distinguished depressive, Gerard
Manley Hopkins. Going to church in these times
seemed tedious and the services long. Other people in
and out of church seemed unreal as if on the other side
of glass. They smiled, they laughed and spoke of
ordinary things, and I felt alien and preoccupied with
self. I felt that God was still there and in time I came to

believe that he was enabling me to suffer, and that it was part of His plan for my life.

I don't think I can believe in the latter now. He was with me, I think, but He couldn't possibly have planned these horrors.

As I have mentioned, I came to draw comfort from others who had suffered similarly. In addition to Hopkins, there were Van Gogh, John Clare and other creative and artistic people. In the pain they were prostrate and lacking the medication available today, yet in the emerging, they created magnificent works. In a much smaller way, I too was creative. I had already written much poetry which much later I published. I loved listening to music, singing, looking at paintings and reading. I had taken part in amateur acting and producing and enjoyed public speaking. I was very sensitive, given to anxiety and entertained massive feelings of guilt. How long I had the seeds of manic depression within me I don't precisely know, but there had been a lot of creativity. Would the former be the price of the latter? In the great and in the ordinary, there would seem to be some sort of connection.

But in the Summer of 1963, I was well, and I was off to Beirut and then to Jerusalem for my course in the Holy Land. The Middle East was incredibly beautiful. It was hot and dusty, full of history, with exposure to Religion deeper than I had before experienced. Seeing places that Christ had seen, and places I had read about, now real, was moving and extraordinary. I was also looking at them below the surface. The entire eight week term was a wonderful experience. Appreciation of my beliefs was also deepened. I was truly enriched. In England, when later I showed my slides and spoke of my adventures, one small boy told his mother that 'Philip had gone to Heaven, and had come back with pictures of it'.

But in all that wonder, in all that Heaven, there was to be a big piece of Hell, not in the places or people, but in what my mind was to do with an innocent experience. I always had an obsessional fear of hurting people and a phobia of causing death even to a tiny creature. If I thought I had hurt someone I would worry about it, so that the blame would increase and I would long for punishment. In time the nightmare would fade to be replaced by something similar.

In Tiberias, while swimming with friends at a lido on the Sea of Galilee, I accidentally kicked a young Israeli boy swimming behind me. I gave it no further thought until that evening when my mind hooked on to the incident and the scenario began to take on frightening proportions, and much later was to re-invent itself in a most alarming hallucination that was to haunt me for about thirty years, triggering off two more enormous breakdowns. It was so tragic that such a wonderful and exciting adventure should be blighted by such horror that was to overshadow such a large proportion of my ministry.

So my mind contrived this tormenting saga. One morning and at home several months later, I woke suddenly with a vivid picture of that Tiberias lido and myself actually beating to death the boy swimmer and then assaulting him sexually. My mind was repulsed. This was not me, so I convinced myself that I had not recalled it before because I had consciously blotted it out at the time, as it was the only way of living with it. I did come to realize that the incident was impossible and not squaring with my nature, my temperament or my conscience. I could not swat a fly or wasp or knowingly tread on a grasshopper. I loved and respected all life. Yet my irrational and bruised mind constantly accused me saying 'You had felt you had killed your rival in the Hall election, so you believed you could quell that guilt by consciously vowing to actually kill someone'.

Yes, I had, I think, entertained this absurd thought occasionally, but to do it was of course out of the question. And for years, I related this internal and tortuous drama to person after person. Every time was so exhausting. I did this to psychiatrists, priests, therapists, friends and family . How I must have tried their patience. Yet no-one complained and no-one said I was mad. All upheld me by their knowledge of me and any spiritual and psychological insights they might have. Once I contacted a friend who was later Dean of Jerusalem and who had been a student with me and a member of the swimming party. He assured me that nothing of the kind could possibly have taken place. My mind would still not be consoled.

Yet all the love, the support, the common sense, the reasoning assurances, could not, save for brief periods, remove the poison which seemed like an insidious serpent in my mind. An overbearing conscience, compounded by a sick mind, continuously appointed the finger of accusation at me. Despite all this I had to continue my studies for my degree, qualify and begin my ministry. The remarkable thing is that I did!

Perhaps the full impact did not dawn until much later, but it must have been beginning before my ordination. Perhaps it was the necessity for hard work and concentration in my finals year that kept disaster at bay. During the first episode and while at home, I had seriously considered abandoning the thought of ordination and returning to librarianship, but I had gone on, and now Finals loomed, and after that a year at Theological College.

I didn't get the class of degree I was expected to get, but all was well in my special subjects Philosophy of Religion and New Testament in Greek, but I could not sufficiently spread a high standard across all the papers. I think there were thirty hours of them in those pre-module days. I was consoled by the award of two prizes, but despite a viva, I could not raise the class of my honours degree. Secretly I blamed my mental problems, but for the present they seemed to be under control, and would continue to be for some time.

After my ordination in Canterbury Cathedral, I went to be Assistant Curate at St. Mark's South Norwood. Here there were additional excessive guilt feelings and self accusation about other matters, like not having fully completed my official papers before being made a deacon. Again this was silly, but my conscience had to be satisfied, like having an inbuilt idol constantly demanding propitiation. I had to be perfect, I had to be absolutely correct, and any hidden imperfection meant to my mind that I was being dishonest even fraudulent.

It was incredible that despite all this self doubting, I was happy in my curacy. Things went very well and I made wonderful friendships with much hospitality. Apart from my activities as curate, I acted in pantomime, and was much involved in youth and children's work. I loved being a priest. If only I could have been easier on myself. I was always ready to help others be accepting of themselves and of other people, but never myself. Always there had to be one 'great crime' I was accusing myself of. I could not convince myself that we are loved and accepted as we are. In my three years in South Norwood the sickness had not gone. It lay dormant under the novelty of ministry, like grey embers of a fire which were temporarily doused.

The choking smoke of depression was just below the surface. I don't even remember the need for medication at this time. It was a good period, a happy time. As I left the parish to move on, I was thirty, still young, very sensitive, vulnerable and with a world of pain still to endure.

So what did depression feel like when it did attack?

It is a monochrome, flat world with something like thick, grey tinted glass between oneself and others. Only people close to one or potential offerers of succour, are acceptable. Medication becomes a lifeline, and when its effects are delayed, it can be tortuous. The pain is not physical but there may be physical appendages. Nonetheless it is searing and goes very deep. The soul aches. Sometimes it abates leaving one numb and disconnected. Sometimes the head feels stuffed with cotton wool and wanting to be banged. The sense of isolation even from carers is immense. Death is a temptation. There is frustration and despair, and the days before a doctor's appointment seem unending. It is horrible, and I doubt that Hell can be worse.

Later I would describe this in poetry. Poetry was to become a 'prize' which the black dog would offer me. But it wasn't a free gift. It was to be paid for in tears,

and in years and years of haunting and debilitating
horror.

CHAPTER 4

SECOND EPISODE.

My ministry continued and led me from my curacy to become the first residential chaplain at a nearby boarding school, the Royal Russell School on the edge of Croydon. It was an exciting and stimulating challenge. I now had my own chapel, small and cosy and with the congregation sitting House of Commons style. I was also resident house tutor for first year boy pupils, aged eleven, and I taught Religious Education for which I designed my own courses. I filled in for additional subjects as required. The staff were a nice lot, very friendly and welcoming. The Second Master was particularly supportive. Generally I enjoyed my time there, preparing many for confirmation, conducting services and being available to any pupil, first in my tiny flat and later when I became housemaster, in more spacious surroundings. As Tutor, I worked closely with the Housemaster and his wife.

They became great friends and colleagues. We got on well and I was happy. Becoming the housemaster was probably a mistake, for although I enjoyed being in charge, it was too much at times on top of being Chaplain. On some matters I began to disagree with the senior staff, and on one occasion with one of the teachers after a very exhausting time with a particular boy whose needs left me drained. The were various house tutors in residence, but this could sometimes be more of a liability than a help. There was no living in matron, so that I was often on my own in charge of the boys at night. I came to dread the sound of not so tiny feet above my sitting room, when I thought they were settled. I would sometimes lose my temper and really fly off the handle in a way probably unacceptable today. So began spasms of guilt again, as I couldn't bear to think that I had in any way hurt any one of my young charges.

Depression, born of exhaustion and guilt began to set in, and one Sunday in my sitting room, and in company with a group of my pupils, there was some silly horseplay which probably went a bit over the top. I began to feel totally wretched. At the same time I developed an obsessional fear of the children catching some disease from the dust in my house. My mind wouldn't rest or accept the possibility that my self accusation was irrational, and my fears exaggerated, not to mention recognizing the emergence of a possible pattern.

I contacted a psychiatrist who had been recommended to me, whose consulting rooms were in London, but who also visited a hospital in Croydon. He proved to be just the man I needed at that time. He first visited me in the school. I think that he diagnosed my problem straight away, but didn't label it. In time I told him of my various fears and anxieties, beginning with the most recent incident. He understood how vulnerable I was. He offered a choice of treatments, anti-depressants or an alternative way, probably lithium as it was to involve regular blood tests. This sounded inconvenient and messy, so I opted for the first suggestion, now, I believe, mistakenly. So for the next twenty years or so, I was never far from a supply of anti-depressants with valium and, when needed, sleeping tablets.   I kept up this private treatment on and off for years, but in time this became spasmodic. This doctor became a safety net and I very much apprcciated this gentle, sympathetic and unstereotyped doctor of the mind. Of all the psychiatrists I would see later, he was by far the best and the most helpful. Considerably later I was to meet two others whom I found appalling, and in my opinion, really unpleasant, who almost seemed to take satisfaction in making matters worse. I suppose that this could have been their method, a kind of shock treatment without electricity, or maybe an odd form of aversion therapy.

So I began to feel reassured and better, and was able to pick myself up and go on, yet while my medication was calming the symptoms, the real causes of my problems must have been continuing to simmer below the surface, in the same way that hidden forces are at work inside a volcano when apparently dormant. One day I do recall feeling so depressed when sitting in the staff room, that I sought an interview with the Head of the Junior school. I remember breaking down and crying. I also wept quite frequently with a friend, the Matron of the neighbouring house. Sometimes I was incapable of doing anything. Some Sundays I would dose myself with valium to get through a service, then I would collapse with relief and released tension. At such times there were no reserves. I sometimes felt desperate and would grasp at any straw. The black dog was constantly at my heels, and sometimes on my back dragging me downwards. When at its worst I didn't want to eat. People seemed distant, and facing a class and trying to teach was a great effort. Running my house was also at times an ordeal. Yet amazingly there were many good times and positive achievements. I recall helping to cope with a severe flu epidemic and taking about ten hours one day to visit every sick pupil. I also helped colleagues in the struggle to keep the school going when it was threatened with closure. Our leader in this inspired us all with his energy and determination, and even he felt enormous strain. The campaign succeeded.

We also held wonderful services as at Christmas and on Remembrance Sunday, while at Harvest Festival the chapel was filled with the most delicious and evocative smells. I recall too an excellent production of the musical 'The Boyfriend' in which I took a part. There was also a very memorable visit by Michael Ramsey, the Archbishop of Canterbury. This took a great deal of careful planning and seemed to go very well. Despite my threatening mental problems, life went on fairly normally, and I knew a lot of happiness. I suppose that the illness was still in its early stages, and I was able to cope.

In 1975 I moved to the Midlands, to Denstone College, a more traditional public school, part of the company of schools forming the Woodard Corporation. There I was Assistant Chaplain, becoming Chaplain a year later.

I came to love this part of the Midlands so near to the Peak District. My brother Charles was living and practicing as a dentist in nearby Derby, and I often visited him for treatment and to see the family. But the black dog came north with me and many were the times when the old guilt and depression returned. I was very foolish not to take my medication regularly but just in emergencies, almost like an addict having a quick fix. At those times, everyday tasks became difficult. I suppose that being surrounded by the ever-present and lively young helped to distract me from the condition. I had great friends, G.D.C. in particular. There was also another colleague M. who seemed entrapped in an 18th century time warp. He called my depressions 'melancholia' for which he would dispense a stiff gin and tonic, very unwise!

One Christmas Day I was staying in my college flat. My parents were staying in Derby with Charles and his family, and I was to join them on Christmas morning for the day. The Vicar of Denstone had asked me to take the early morning service in the parish church. At some point before or after the service and in the vestry when I was alone, I was suddenly overwhelmed by a feeling of complete loneliness and self pity, coupled with a sense of guilt and depression. The fact of it being Christmas Day was probably the catalyst or trigger. I broke down and wept uncontrollably. Why no-one was there to see me, I have no idea, but I was able to compose myself, and on with the motley. One day I might return to that church and see my dampened signature in the register.

Depression is something that separates us from normality. It is as if one is on an isolated island and the sky above is always black and threatening. You see and hear other people, but at a distance, and they cannot know what it feels like. To all outward appearances you will look normal unless they know you very well indeed. One goes through the motions as far as possible, but even one's own words and actions seem remote as if spoken through cotton wool or in an echo chamber. It's unreal and yet painfully real at the same time. When with people, one craves to be alone. But being alone only brings brief relief, for the thoughts go on. If any action is attempted, it is very exhausting.

Only night and a sleeping aid bring total relief, but sometimes sleeplessness or early morning waking with cold or hot sweats and an onrush of anxiety removes all ability to rest. In any case, very early morning or just early morning would open the floodgates and the fears would be enormous. I had no desire to get up, so I would reassure my frightened self that after a few hours, I would be climbing back into bed again when oblivion would again bring relief. If I could, I found that getting up and doing something would slightly reduce the level of anxiety. The spiral of fatigue was debilitating.

There were also manic times, when again sleep was elusive. I would get out of bed and tackle some work like the preparation of a major service. I would work for hours in the middle of the night until all was done.

I sometimes thought of confessing the crimes I had imagined, or even of going to the police, but this would have caused unnecessary trouble, for I knew in my more rational moments that my fears were not facts. I contemplated suicide, but I knew I couldn't do it, especially because of the harm it would do to my mother. I had probably already caused her much anxiety. It was unthinkable to cause her any more distress. Besides I was a coward. Every possible way of ending my life filled me with dread. In any case I might not succeed, which might leave me in a more distressing state. Also there was my faith. My life and the life of others was sacred. It is just that my mind screamed out for relief and for the stopping of incessant and accusing thoughts. I envied the very old and the dead.

And still I went on, rarely taking time off, getting on with my duties, often very public ones in front of the whole school. The two successive headmasters didn't particularly like me, not because of my inner turmoil which was largely hidden, but perhaps because any school chaplain had too much exposure in their school. Also I had an inbuilt antipathy to people in authority and could be very critical, In my career I was not a particularly humble person, and though inwardly I was accusing myself, yet I believed in my competence, and loved being liked.

It was also while I was at Denstone that I first became involved in broadcasting and the B.B.C. I had volunteered a chapel service to Radio Stoke. This accordingly was recorded to celebrate one of the Queen's anniversaries, probably her 25th. This led to my taking a course in broadcasting followed by broadcasts, both live and recorded, for Radio Stoke. I also did a week's 'Thought for the day' for Radio 4,which I recorded in Manchester. Thereafter wherever I was, I made occasional broadcasts right up to the present day. This again shows that it is possible to do other things and not allow the illness to swamp everything, except of course in the dreaded episodes.

Denstone was generally a happy part of my life. It is extraordinary that though my mind was so often in turmoil and at times, in despair, I could be happy. It may be, that in part, these residential communities cocoon a person, giving a sense of security and protection. I was often in pain, yet for the most part I lived within buildings largely cut off from the outside, so to an extent, I felt safe.

Then came the big move. The senior school of this whole group of Woodard schools is Lancing College on the Sussex coast between Brighton and Worthing. I had visited Lancing in 1978 as a representative of Denstone, at the great service to dedicate the new West window by the Archbishop of Canterbury in the presence of the Prince of Wales. The position of Chaplain of Lancing became vacant. Encouraged by a previous chaplain and a Provost of the Midlands division, I applied and was interviewed. As I stood in the amazingly high chapel, the 4th highest church in the country, I couldn't believe that I should ever be appointed. It was a short time later, and while revisiting St.George's, Jerusalem, that the call came through. The Head of Rugby school and soon to be Head of Lancing phoned, offering me the appointment. I was elated. The skies had cleared, and if there was a cloud left, it was numbered 'nine'! The remaining time at Denstone was a mixture of sadness at leaving so many friends with the joy of anticipation.

In January 1982, I arrived at Lancing in ice and snow, and climbed the stone steps of the Masters' Tower to my flat in the eaves. The bathroom which was cold and Spartan, was shared with others including a very taciturn biologist. Shaving in adjacent basins was a strange experience, one I had not known since student days. While I was at Lancing these facilities were considerably modernised.

For some reason I felt intimidated and unsure in my early days at Lancing. On the first day of term, I was so afraid that I couldn't face the common room at morning break. This irrational distress was in itself a sign. Yet here, as everywhere there were kind and generous colleagues, some of them schoolmasters in the old mould, some young and confident, and most of them very academic. I missed my first lesson completely, having misread the timetable, but was given another class instead! I began to feel better, but never did feel comfortable with the 6th form General Divinity, a cause of much anxiety. Some pupils thought it voluntary and stayed away, then had to be chased up. Most classes went well, but there seemed to be a culture of unkindness which some pupils and colleagues suffered. This unpleasantness certainly added to my worries account. I was however inspired by the grandeur of the chapel, and in all modesty, I think I rose to many an occasion there, and was happy to enter into its dignity.

The first term passed, but returning for the Summer term, I felt increasingly uneasy. Something menacing was stirring. What set it off was a kind word from the Head in a college news letter, saying how much everyone had come to trust me. But I felt guilty of so much and considered myself a fraud and completely unworthy of anyone's trust. The old negative feelings began to come back, and I rapidly slowed down. I sank lower and lower and felt terrible, and very lonely. How I longed for the small fields and hills of Staffordshire. A kind of homesickness became part of a horrible stark illness. With an old prescription, I obtained a quantity of valium and tried to numb the pain. At some point during the term, I took the train to London to see my Croydon psychiatrist who gave me more medication. Then one day I came to a full stop. I slumped into an armchair. I phoned the Head, and within minutes, his wife, a kind and well-meaning person, plucked me out of the Tower, and I was installed in the Head's house for a 'complete rest'. I collapsed into this comfort and relished their genuine welcome. I was isolated from the school save for a few visitors. Yet there was still the blackness of despair and a total lack of energy. It took me ages to get up in the morning and then I was done for.

Eventually it was agreed that I should return to the school and to my flat, but as I entered the Tower, there were two boys in the quad. I heard one say to the other 'There's Psycho'. Thereafter that was my nick-name amongst the pupils. I think the name was mostly used without malice, but accompanied by sly hisses as I passed by, it was a repeated reminder of my unstable state, even though invisible to others. The name of course was used long after its origins were understood.

Most pupils and all colleagues were kind, understanding and supportive, and before long many pupils were choosing me for their tutor.

I cannot recall any specific medical help at this time though the school doctor was to be very understanding when needed.

The term should have been lovely, as Summer in Sussex was beautiful, and there were plenty of outdoor events with Founder's day as their climax. But before long I had another major collapse. The earlier event had been just a rumble compared with ferocity of the horrific storm to come. Once again I crashed, once again back to the Head's house. But despite their best efforts, I got worse and sunk lower and lower. I was getting lost in a very thick fog, and everyone and everything were receding fast. I had no energy or willpower left. I did not want to belong. The Assistant Chaplain came and anointed me. The Bishop of Lewes, then Vice Provost visited and was sympathetic. But they were losing me. Something had to be done and fast.

It was arranged that I should be admitted to the Psychiatric Hospital in Chichester as a voluntary patient. I was desperate for help, so all my fears and prejudices about such institutions had to be repressed. This place was to be the first of three such institutions I was to experience. None was to help, but rather, it seemed to me, they would push me deeper into my private despair. I longed to be at home, but at this point I didn't think that my family knew.   I was trying to cushion my mother for as long as possible. In any case everyone by now seemed to be on another planet.

Before me lay a degrading abyss. I could never be the same person again.

Poems below followed by chapter 5.

BREAKDOWN

There is a blackness darker than deepest shade,
Which eating into the soul drags it downwards.
Ever downwards into depths painful and alone,

Sapping life's energies and despite oneself makes void all hope.

In it the mind cries 'Why?' while no answer comes.

Into these searing pits I have lately walked,

Visited before but on ledges higher than the mists below.

Here I have wandered glimpsing others in this hell;

Hero souls sitting solitary and vacantly brooding,

Waiting to be rescued, lifted from the valley floor.

Swirling mists and sightless fogs capturing the mind,

And closing, sealing off all doors save seeing

Others walking in the light and envious of their joy.

Body and mind torn apart severed by the mood,

Only night brings hope, the morning shattering fragile dreams,

And dark despair returns to cover all beneath

This dreadful savage pall so black

And unlike night, unlit by moon or any kind of light.

1982 (from 'Deal Pier and other poems.)

AND IT WAS NIGHT.

Evening contains the haunted reveries of tale and play.
Sunset and fantasy trade on thoughts, imaginings of
day.
The mind is open to the grey suggestions,
And daydreams lay the ghosts who walk.

Night erases memories of what was done the day
before.
Darkness and dreams blot out the thoughts of
yesterday.
The mind can only cope with what it comprehends,
And nightmares store the black remainder.

Morning returns the cold and stark proportions of all
life.
Sunrise and reality isolate and freeze meanderings of
the night.

The mind is stilled and looses all excitement,

And pragmatics stifle reaching beyond death.

                    1987 (from 'Deal Pier

and other poems.')

CHAPTER 5

THE PIT AND AFTERMATH. 1982-1990.

Apart from the major symptoms, other effects of the illness gathered. Basically they formed an overbearing obsessive scrupulosity. As a boy, when my parents were out, even just at the end of the road, I would lie awake in bed, anxious to hear their key in the lock. When they did return which was never very late, I would go through a ritual of saying 'thank you' one hundred times. If I had been God, I would have turned off early! Then much later there was my irrational fear of the dust at the Royal Russell school. It was just ordinary everyday dust which is present in every home, but for me it became a matter of life or death. To this was added the compulsion to remember every 'significant' detail on a car journey, and at home I would relive the entire journey, recalling the details and ticking them off on a piece of paper. This made car journeys totally exhausting. I would do the same for ordinary events in the day and for conversations however inconsequential. Every tiny detail assumed exaggerated proportions, and if I couldn't remember one of them, I would be frantic. Yet at the same time, I was achieving and doing my job as well as my unforgiving standards demanded, I was the slave of an unbalanced conscience with a mind that was losing control.

The crash was inevitable.

And what was happening now was a new experience. I was sliding downhill in a big way, and in an institution I never imagined I would be in except as a visitor. Yes, I had visited patients in the past, but me, never! Where I was, was brought home to me speedily. My personal possessions were taken from me into 'safe keeping'. My medication was likewise removed. As I lay in bed that night, the mattress covered in plastic sheeting, I began to question for the first time what God was doing. Oddly too I recall thinking,' Well I'll never be a bishop now.' This is almost humorous looking back, yet it betrays a certain arrogance and an inflated belief in my own abilities. As if ambition mattered when my mind lay in shatters. The sleeping pill took a long time to work, and the it seemed immediately, I was awakened by a young man in the opposite bed screaming uncontrollably. So I was in hospital, a strange and austere place, no doubt a former workhouse, with strange and broken people sleeping in the same room, with no personal property and no family or friends near. My future hopes and ambitions were in tatters and I had no hope left. I slept fitfully. Not even the night was bringing consolation.

As the day came and hospital life dragged on, I became increasingly desperate.

I was determined to leave as soon as possible. I telephoned Charles, not wanting to upset my parents and begged to be brought out. Poor man, he was running his dental practice in Derby. He also had a wife and three young boys to care for. But I could only see my own needs. I think that soon after I spoke to my parents. The doctor assessing me chain smoked his way through the interview in a smelly and dingy room. Soon after leaving him, I felt compelled to see him again about something which seemed enormously important. He was brutally dismissive, uninterested and irritated. That was the level of psychiatric care from him, but then he was seeing people like me and worse all day. No doubt it would get to anyone. I was heartbroken too because I had no razor and couldn't shave, or so I thought. I collapsed onto a chair outside the doctor's room and wept loudly. I was in total despair. I was full of self pity and felt completely cut off. A kind nurse sat beside me and comforted me. She produced my shaving kit and I was able to shave. I felt better for that.

I did try by walking in the grounds and by talking to other patients. The problem was that they tended to gather around me and I couldn't help giving them some pastoral care, perhaps unwittingly. It was instinctive. Yet I knew I shouldn't, and that it was tiring. I was enjoying my contact with certain patients in particular and I felt less isolated. I again spoke to Charles who was by this time negotiating with the staff to collect me and take me to his home in Derby. It was on the understanding that I would seek medical help there.

At no time do I recall a hospital doctor talking to me
about my illness and giving some kind of diagnosis.
I suppose I was in hospital on that occasion for no
longer that three days, but it seemed much longer. I was
so pleased and relieved to see my brother. So we left
that place of so much sadness. We stopped at Lancing
for lunch with the Head and his wife, and we went
to my flat to pack some things. I felt so much better
already. On the journey north, I unburdened myself to
Charles, telling him of my imaginings and of the Holy
Land 'event'. He was remarkably accepting, for it must
have been his first encounter with chronic mental
illness, and he was letting me come into his home and
live with his family.
Yet at the time it was to be my salvation. My first meal
with them that evening was like a banquet, in contrast
to the hospital. Also there was the luxury of sleeping in
my own room with my own wash basin.Sheer bliss.
Charles' wife, Sally was a physiotherapist, and Charles
being a dentist, meant that their care was enhanced by
medical insight. I was to be occupied, have plenty of

rest and good food, with a regular walk every afternoon. I also read quantities of books. I went to see an understanding local doctor who arranged my medication. At weekends Charles would drive us all out into the countryside.

Generally my thinking became more positive and I began to see a future. But how could I be accepted back at Lancing? As we passed village churches on our drives, I considered abandoning the thought of being a school chaplain and applying for a parish job. The school kept in touch, and it was very clear that I was wanted back. But to return was still a daunting prospect, as my illness and its nature would surely be known to all.

Five weeks later I did return, and it was arranged that I would stay with the Assistant Chaplain and his equally caring wife. They were so kind and patient just as my brother and Sally had been, and before long I made a visit to the Staff Common Room during a morning break. I need not have worried. For everyone was so welcoming and kind. My head still felt like cotton wool and I felt insecure and fragile, but I had made a first step back to normality. It was agreed, very sensibly, that I would resume normal life in the school, for the last week of term, so that starting again in September would be that much easier. I took part in chapel one Sunday evening, I taught, I met pupils and colleagues. I did it and came through.

On the chapel sacristans' outing, a very strange thing happened. I had been feeling fairly subdued and certainly not on top form. It must have been a Sunday. After a picnic we sat by the river prior to returning to the school for Evensong. Suddenly like a rush of adrenalin, I was in a totally different mood and full of vitality. My entire being took off. I thought it was a miracle and that I was cured. I challenged some of the pupils to a run back to the minibus, and not only did I run, I skipped and jumped. It was certainly a high, but as yet I did not understand the nature of my illness, and the term 'manic' had not been explained.
But something in my brain must have triggered change of mood and feeling. I had gone into overdrive and it

was terrific. Back at the school I was still feeling buoyant, and said that I would take Evensong. My being there must have taken many people by surprise, including the Head who looked across to me in an encouraging manner when we sang the line of a hymn,' health to the sick in mind'. I cannot recall any immediate sequel except of course that the elation didn't last, but I suppose it must have helped in my short resumption of duties.

I spent most of my summer holidays quietly with my parents. The Head invited me to crew on a boat belonging to him and his brother. We sailed to the Channel Islands and to France. I thoroughly enjoyed it and the people I met. It was a wonderful experience and a real tonic.

My return to the school in September went quite well, and I returned quickly to the routine. Just occasionally the depression returned for short periods and I relied on medication, albeit in fits and starts. I remember one morning in my time at Lancing being overcome by depression, becoming virtually immobile for a time. A much liked tutorial pupil of mine had been killed in the south of France. I was deeply affected by this, as were many others. This was probably something of a trigger to my mood, as I was preparing his memorial service for the following Sunday. I wept copiously while John the Assistant Chaplain, comforted me.

There was another occasion that I particularly remember. It was a very empty Saturday afternoon. My mood darkened perceptibly and remorselessly. I was alone. I had no medication, and I was soon in what was virtually a state of collapse. The school doctor was not available, but the sanatorium nurse offered me some company. She realized how desperate I was becoming, and eventually managed to obtain something which would take the edge off the syptoms, so I scraped through.

It was while I was at Lancing that a friend invited me to accompany him on a holiday in Sri Lanka. It wasn't long before I began to feel very ill and would gaze out to sea, thinking I would never see my family again. I was taken to a doctor and given medication. When that ran out, I went to Chemists where valium was in ample supply, sold cheaply over the counter. On a trip up country I was overdosing and my body went in to spasms. It was frightening, and so far from home. As an emergency, my time there was curtailed and a flight was arranged. I was so relieved to be back in England and immediately I began to feel better.

There was also the time when the Head came down heavily on me for something quite innocent involving a parent who had given permission to me to take her son for a short bargain break to Paris. She then changed her mind, and reported the matter to the Head. I was shocked by this turn of events, quarrelled with the Head, broke down in front of the boy's housemaster, and left for the summer holidays without attending the usual festivities. The Head's part in this didn't square with the way in which he and his wife had shown me so much kindness with patience and understanding a few years earlier. When he left for Malawi where Lancing was twinned with another school, I felt somewhat exposed and being unable to resolve the situation between us which was frustrating. He had left behind a very long letter which he had sent to the Provost who saw me and interviewed me.

He seemed to assume that I was a homosexual. The evidence was without foundation, to say the least, uncertain, and I had done nothing. The Head was no doubt at the end of his tether. My poor old mind felt battered and bruised, and tested, yet though I was fed up, I was oddly not at that time particularly depressed. Even the black dog was subdued by what I perceived to be an unfair attack on my integrity. At the beginning of the next term I met the Head over tea. He was pleasant, constructive and positive, but I knew that He was concerned about recent 'highs' and really wanted me to move on. This was but A stay of execution.

So what were these highs like?

I can remember three incidents, but there were probably more. The first was the one I have already described on the sacristans' outing. Another was when the Provost was visiting one of my classes, and I suggested that he be a 'pupil' in the class.

I felt really on top form. My words of teaching flowed and I spoke rapidly and excitedly. I fired question after question at the poor man who blinked at the speed with which the questions came, sometimes not allowing answers. I don't know whether he knew what was happening, and at the time I wasn't aware of anything wrong. I only knew that I felt very happy and blissfully unaware that I was acting oddly. Another occasion was at a special dinner in the staff dining room Various dignitaries were there from the school governing body including a bishop. I reveled in such occasions. I was not born into social grace and elegance, albeit brought up well, but I took to all social occasions like a duck to water. No-one in any hierarchy was a problem, and the more distinguished a person was, the more I glowed. I regarded such events as a challenge and a deserved privilege. On this particular occasion, I was speaking rapidly and excitedly. a true sign, I now know, of 'mania' at least for me. I also felt myself to be amusing, as people seemed to be laughing and enjoying my repartee. I loved to be listened to and I loved the resulting laughter. But later I was told that I had shocked the Chairman by something I had said. Their laughter perhaps had just been politeness, but I had mistaken it for enjoyment, food for a clown's vanity. I was a fool who longed to show sweetness, but it was turning bitter.

So my crimes were 'errors of judgement', and my condition would eventually be identified as 'manic depression'. I did not need to be censored. I needed to be helped. I did not need to be judged. I needed accurate diagnosis. To a discerning eye I was supplying enough symptoms for right recognition and treatment. Yet the volcano in my brain would go on unrecognized for some time, and would seriously erupt once more before someone would spot what was wrong and bring me relief and hope at last.

ALONE

Alone,

I am alone,

Subject to thoughts that do disturb

And haunt the stillness.

Contemplative of things that will not curb

The mind's alarms, till less

Of peace and more of fear is born

To me who am alone.

Alone.

Alone,

I am alone,

Exposed to penetrating beams of light

That find me waiting,

Unlike as when in company, when sight

Of others close the gate. Bring

hope and quiet expectancy

To me who am alone.

I am alone.

Alone.

Alone,

I am alone.

No more afraid though anguish was at home

And laid me low.

Now neither threats nor fears to come

Can harm. Tree blow

Of Calvary must be far worse

For Him who was alone.

I am alone,

So we are one

Alone,

With terror gone.

1988 (from 'Deal Pier and other poems)

FENCE

A man has built a fence

Blocking views of field and sea

Closing me in on the pretence

Of improvement for his unborn child, while we

Must stand on tiptoe, or sense

Loses sight that would be free.

Another man has built a fence

Stifling and strangling what would be me,

Urging on my spirit, silence,

And diminishing restrictions to be

Less than I was whence

Blighted seed now grown to tree.

A man has built a fence.

Not God who made me

To know laughter, love, with licence

To grow so tall, dangling on a knee,

But now a man to innocence

Restored and filled with glee.

Though man has built a fence,
Keeping me constrained, a prisoner to be,
'll use it as a means to rest upon, and thence
To grow and go on growing and see
The barrier now mounting block, hence
Climbing step to Thee.

                    1988 (from 'Deal Pier and other
        poems')

SLEEP AND RISING

Restless and sleepless were the hours of night,

Comfortless stretches in the black.

Hour filled stretches without sight

Turning upon a comfortable rock.

Then suddenly asleep and for an hour or more

A deepening of the night.

And then the morning kind and bright,

As consciousness returns, and light

Visits the late troubled bed and opens new day's door.

This and every night a kind of dying

Which following on a troubled life

Brings back unconsciousness, a timeless lying

Still in the space between living and rising'

When the spirit severed from the shell

Puts restlessness behind, bypassing strife and Hell,

Goes through the new day's door and lives.

1992 (from 'Deal Pier and other

      poems')

CHAPTER 6

THIRD EPISODE   1990.

Before the next showdown with my mind, a friend,
interested in psychoanalysis put
me in touch with an analyst in Brighton, a woman who
had been recommended to him. I saw her once a week
for an hour. It was an interesting and very helpful
experience. I would do most of the talking with an
occasional interjection with her. When I asked
questions, her responses were always most reassuring.
It was sometimes like a confessional, and I had
complete confidence in her. She was sympathetic and
always professional. She commented on my dreams
which I would bring to her. She was particularly helpful
with what she said about my obsessional thinking. All
in all I think she was encouraging me not to be so hard
on myself and to come to terms with sexuality and
other basics, but also to take responsibility in a
measured way when appropriate. I was totally frank

with her, because we got on well and because of her professionalism. Oddly I could never imagine her in a supermarket, and whereas my words flowed in her consulting room, I would have been struck dumb meeting her in Tesco's!

I had previously tried Hypnotherapy with a doctor in Eastbourne. It was a strange undertaking. He explained that it was not sleep. I would remain conscious but completely relaxed and free of inhibitions. I came out of most sessions feeling quite refreshed, and would bounce back to the school feeling re-invigorated, but I doubt that we got to grips with my problems. He was helpful in the short term. Even my psychoanalyst could only help so far. I think that both kinds of therapy work in the belief that the mind when more fully understood can be its own healer. I would never discourage anyone from seeking help in these ways, but depending on the nature of the illness, other ways may provide a more effective cure, or at least should complement.

At Lancing a new Provost was appointed and installed, and within a short time, he suggested to me that I consider 'giving something to parish ministry'. Clearly the Head and he had been talking. The Provost had no knowledge of school chaplaincy as far as I could judge. Also it was apparent that I was liked and respected by my colleagues, and, I think, by most of the pupils. I knew that this is where I belonged. I pondered the suggestion for a week, and responded by saying that I would move on if he could find a parish between Lancing and Dover where my mother was living, also that it should be near the sea and have a school. As if by magic, the Provost produced from his pocket a piece of paper with details of two rural parishes in East Sussex that fitted my requirements. I visited the villages incognito with a Matron friend. I liked what I saw and told the Bishop of Lewes that I was interested in going further. I was interviewed by the four churchwardens. Two of them were somewhat formidable. One of these, a woman judge spoke with authority but also with some humour. The other, smaller and sharp as a starling, asked me among her questions whether I was a homosexual. Taken aback and not being entirely sure of the answer, I said 'no'. I now reflect that I could have been somewhat annoyed at this intrusion on my privacy. After all it was to be some years before the subject became a burning issue in the Church of England. In any case I believe that a priest's sexuality should not affect his ability in any aspect of his ministry. What matters is whether he is faithful or promiscuous, whatever his leanings. My lack of sexual experience was perhaps the more concerning shortcoming.

Eventually and after an overwhelming send off from Lancing, I went to the Rectory in Ninfield and to the two parishes of Ninfield and Hooe. My mother, widowed since 1984,together with her close friend and helper, Cyril, assisted me in settling in. The Induction in Ninfield was in a packed church including pupils and staff from Lancing. The Bishop in his sermon told my new parishioners to respect my celibacy and give me space to settle. This was surprising as I had never labeled myself celibate even though I was living the celibate life, and as for giving me space, I badly needed to see people after my crowded flat in Lancing. The reception following the service, in the church primary school was a very happy event. Soon after, Mother and Cyril returned to East Kent, and I was now truly on my own and at the 'deep end'.

So it was that my flat at school which had been frequently full of young life was exchanged for a spacious house and garden, at that time very empty and silent, and in a community where I was a total stranger. The young who had filled my previous ministry were thus far non-existent and now most of the parishioners seemed very old. Lancing's chapel had been frequently full, some six hundred or more. On my first Sunday Evensong I looked from the pulpit onto about six elderly pates. I had swapped a choir of fifty for empty choir stalls, and the pupils in the school were not bright teenagers but small children from four upwards. What had the Provost been thinking of? Why had no-one intervened in this appointment?   And yet, though trouble lay ahead, eventually I would come to love my parishes very much, and I would come to know peace of mind such as I had not known for a very long time.

A month after my Induction, and at the beginning of October, a mental storm more vicious than I had known before broke over me. It was Monday morning, my day off. I was just sitting in my study, and in utter despair, Space and time seemed a total vacuum. I was as low as ever, and I knew that this was no passing mood. In all this blackness I felt I couldn't be alone. I went to the doctor's surgery, and there I saw Alan, a member of the congregation. I asked if I could go to his home with him, which I did. He was perhaps a bit uncertain, but when we arrived, his wife Molly seemed to understand, and I was made welcome. That day I was fed and cared for by them. That afternoon, the Rural Dean arrived and suggested that I go to a nearby Christian Home of Healing.

I do know, that for many, this place was very helpful, In deep countryside with a lovely garden, the home provided gentle hospitality, spiritual support and much T.L.C. It has a beautiful chapel and a staff who tried very hard to help. At first I believed that the Warden, a priest would really help. But to me he seemed out of his depth and incapable of recognizing that I was ill beyond his resources, So I became increasingly desperate. My depression became vice-like with no remission. I grasped at the offer of exorcism. I claimed that I had been released. I was anxious to be better but also to please. There was much rejoicing. But it was self-delusion, and I sank even deeper.

I felt that the Warden was beginning to lose interest, and was getting tetchy. My friend John the assistant chaplain at Lancing was contacted, and he kindly came to see me. We sat in the garden and the flood gates opened. There was some discussion between John and the Warden. The latter emerged looking very displeased. I had begged John to get me to a doctor. I felt at the time that The Warden felt threatened.

As the Warden drove me back to Ninfield where an appointment with my G.P. had been made, he rebuked me for speaking to John, and hoped that I had not said critical things about him. I was broken and felt suicidal, but this supposed man of God bullied me, and went on to accuse me of undermining his work.

I saw my doctor. He decided that with my consent, I should go to the local psychiatric hospital, and this I was then taken to. Anything and anywhere to receive help, was all I could think of. So in the darkness I arrived at another institution for the mentally ill. Perched on a small cliff above the sea, it might have been beautiful, but there was nothing of the picture postcard here. This hospital was stark, bleak and it seemed, unwelcoming. Yet who cared? I was free of the Home of Healing and its Warden!

A kindly nurse looked after me on my first evening. For that first night, I actually had my own room, spartan but peaceful and secure. The next morning the impact of where I was, hit me. A grim looking nurse, who looked like the archetype of a female prison camp warder, told me that I could only use the toilet with the door wide open. This was because apparently I was regarded as a suicide risk. I was heart broken. I had been stripped of my pride and ambition, and now I was to be robbed of all dignity. My suicide threat had been cry for help and attention, but I suppose they couldn't take risks. We compromised and I agreed to leave the door ajar.

The few days I was there were occupied in talking to some of the other patients, eating unappetizing food, and doing jigsaw puzzles. Again I was to meet some very brave and lovely people, but some were so traumatized that they just stood in the middle of the room staring into space. I wondered whether it was good to mix breakdown sufferers with the extremely ill, but perhaps in mental health, this is a mistaken distinction. My mother and Cyril visited me, and as they were leaving, there appeared two well meaning parishioners clutching a copy of 'The History of Hooe church'.

I pleaded with the doctors to be allowed home, and a psychiatrist said it would be all right provided I sought medical help. I was elated and probably went into manic mode. I know that at my last lunch there, I upset one of the staff dispensing food, who muttered something discouraging.

The night before I left the hospital, a young man was admitted. He was a university student, and had tried to throw himself from an upstairs window. He seemed extremely manic as he spoke very rapidly and often he didn't make sense. I befriended him and tried to be sympathetic. I even helped him prepare for bed, but of course respected his need for space and privacy.

The next day I was collected by my mother and Cyril, and went to my cottage where my mother was living, in the Kent coast village of St. Margaret's at Cliffe. I was so happy to be out of hospital, and for a time things went well. Mother and Cyril were supportive, kind and helpful. I remember being visited by Cyril's great grandchildren. They were four lovely children all with blond hair. They sat on a sofa, speechless and just looking at me. They were sweet, but we might have been on different planets.

Depression began to increase and it became almost disabling. My mother was extremely brave, but it must have been very difficult for her. I was very thankful for her company and was able to talk. One Saturday lunchtime I was in despair. There was no deeper and darker place for my head to go. It was near tangible. I was in a black cul-de-sac and was truly desperate. In a recent emergency the family doctor had prescribed, but I noticed the dosage on the label was much in excess of what it should have been, so the drug was recalled. Something else was then prescribed, but soon after beginning to take it, my jaws went into alarming spasms. An emergency doctor was sent for. He injected me with an antidote, causing the spasms to subside. It was very frightening, and when I went to bed that night, I was exhausted. The spasms began again but were arrested by the sleeping pill, and so I slept.

We tried returning to the parishes, and I attempted to take an Evensong. Mother and Cyril visited the Rectory several times, and on one occasion I began to feel awful, so they came again. I was prostrate. One of the churchwardens came and I confessed my despair. She told me that a colleague's daughter had gone to a nearby private hospital. She generously said that she would finance me if I wanted to go. Soon it was arranged and we drove over for my admission.

The hospital looked like a stately home, white and classical, in beautiful parkland and just outside a village. It had been built in the 19th Century, and its first patients had been clergymen. My room was very comfortable with en suite facilities. There was no problem about razors here! There was a comfortable lounge, a gym and a dining room, an art room, consulting rooms and sitting rooms for group sessions. The meals were well prepared, colourful and carefully presented. For my first meal, I sat opposite a young woman who said little, ate little and was clearly upset. She was suffering from M.E. ,a condition I have never really understood, and I have since known a number of brave sufferers.

The next morning was my assessment by my assigned psychiatrist. We didn't hit it off from the start. He was abrupt, at times sarcastic and appeared disinterested. I poured it all out. I was well rehearsed. I guess he'd heard it all before. Some said that he was a good doctor. I had little evidence to support this. Hospital psychiatrists and I don't click! He prescribed another cocktail of tablets.

We patients spent a lot of time talking to one another. I went jogging every morning before breakfast. We were given exercises in the gym, and I would do additional exercises there. We had group sessions, and once I was rebuked for saying too much, or possibly the wrong thing! I went to art classes and much was read into my very poor painting. We went on guided walks, and as Christmas approached, we were taken to Tunbridge Wells. The shopping trip felt awful, the decorations in shops and streets adding to the pathos. On one of our excursions we went into a park and I suddenly became manic and started running around, talking excitedly to the others. Such episodes were very exhausting.

That afternoon I was to visit the local Vicar. He had earlier brought me Holy Communion at the hospital. He was pleasant and welcoming which made one particular comment of his that much more surprising. During our conversation he said 'Depression does not bring glory to God'. I should have asked 'Did crucifixion?', but I was so taken aback. This man was respected in the diocese and probably popular in his parish, but pastorally to me, he was something of a disaster. I had so far met two very insensitive priests in my illness.

I remember well November the 5th when we were all invited to a bonfire party, but I didn't go. I also remember another patient attaching himself to me, and he would tell me his problems in great detail. We became friends, but I was gently rebuked by the staff for getting too involved for I too was ill and shouldn't be strained. I recall unenjoyable sessions with my assigned doctor and also kindly hardworking nurses. I do remember another doctor who was very serious, but patient and comforting. I could speak to him and did. What upset me about some of the treatment I had received from hospital doctors over the years, was that I was shown so little respect. I also was a professional man, qualified in my field, experienced and adult. My illness changed none of that. But the psychiatrists particularly, were largely blinkered to this. I seemed to lose all status when in their care. I did not expect to be treated differently from the other patients. They all deserved this kind of consideration. In my own pastoral and hospital visiting, I have always tried to respect each individual whatever the situation.

I asked to be discharged, and this my psychiatrist reluctantly permitted. In any case I had this right as a voluntary patient. I really had been so very homesick. One Sunday afternoon earlier, when Mother, Cyril and my aunt had come over, and following their departure, I was in a terrible state and my depression deepened. The nurse could give me no medication without a doctor, so I just had to grin and bear it. Gradually the mood lifted a little, and the routine resumed.

So I could leave.

I can't recall whether we went back to Ninfield at that time. I do know that the year was moving on, and it was now doubtful that I could do anything in my parishes at Christmas. The decision was made, and I returned to St.Margaret's and to Wells cottage.

Then something marvelous happened.

I think it began with a visit from a psychiatric nurse, arranged by the local surgery. He recommended that I undergo a short course of E.C.T., electric convulsive therapy. This form of treatment is, I think, not so much in favour now, and didn't suit everyone who underwent it, but I was willing to try anything to feel better, and I was concerned that my mother should benefit. I felt that I was dragging her down though she never complained. So it began. A hospital car came and regularly took Mother and me to yet another psychiatric hospital. This particular one had been the stuff of schoolboy humour as it was our local mental asylum. I had visited a patient there some years before. It was big,Victorian, forbidding and has since closed down.

I had no idea what to expect. On the day of our first visit it was frosty and cold, but inside the reception room, it was bright, warm and colourful and festooned with Christmas decorations. A warm and beaming nurse showed us to our seats, took details, explained the procedure and left. In a short time I was led to the treatment room. A young doctor asked me to lie on a bed. I was made secure and then given an anaesthetic. I'm glad I never saw or knew exactly what happened, but I guess it would not have been a pretty sight. I recovered consciousness and rejoined my mother for a cup of tea and a biscuit. I had been told that I might not notice any change for several sessions. I was due to have four. I was also aware that for some people it seemed to have little effect.

Remarkably I began to feel an improvement after my first treatment, and I looked forward as each session came round. I am sure that the kindness of the staff contributed to my recovery. They were all wonderful, in contrast to some I had met before. So I responded and began to look forward, for the first time, to Christmas.

IN SOLITARY

In the space between people
Is a void and loveless place,
Where talk is to oneself and to my
Face reflected back from glass.
There are the pets and disembodied television voices
Attached to glamorous faces,
Familiar but unknown,
Talking to cameras and technicians.
These do not relieve the empty spaces,
Save for the fleeting seconds of ideas sown.

There is the telephone, but it spells distant places.
There is the window and the figures are apart
And unconnected.
For them I am not head or heart.

'Loneliness is in the mind.' Not true.
Its taste is in the air, its breath inhaled.
If solitary is peace, the other railed

In arid openness and on my fate impaled.

There are the treasured times of being

I with one just here,

When voices cease and all is calm,

But how the lonely longs for someone near,

The common pairing lot of man brings balm.

1995 from ('The plague of 2001

and other poems'.)

GONE BEFORE

This earth is but a place of sadness
Bathed in death.
For where the feet of present people step,
There others long since dead have walked,
Breathing and living, laughed and wept.
Now the long gone dead who have been everywhere
Then talked,
And for a time was immortality,
But soon and always really, knew it was mortality.
No matter who, all have to die,
While we look out as layers of those before us tie
Idealism down to what we know but care to shun,
Crowding out the requiem sound , drowning the tearful
with a tonne
Of artificial noise, as tinsel covers oaken chest,
And we see present living as the best
Of worlds, while all around us are remains of lives
Who disbelieved in death save for the countless cries
Of others,' Never me.'

So layer on layer once living breathing souls

Make carpets for our feet, while bowls

Of ash and charnel contents just below the sod

Make passages and paths for spirits meeting God.

So does our world seem full of life,

Yct all's illusion and death does populate this knife-

Edge of my brief existence.

2000 (from 'The plague
of 2001 and other poems.')

ME OR NOT TO BE?

I am respectable, living politely, full
Of noble thoughts and good intentions.
The public face of me is nice and never mentions
Anything that's wrong.

My public image is intact,
Of good report and if it lacked,
I would endeavor to make up,
And if offending, fill the cup
With my apologies, lest tarnish
Stains my reputation.

Yet there is part of me
I know and would set free,
A part which seeks excess,
Painting red the town no less
Because it's there and looks so drab.
This is the other side of everyone.
Careless of common approbation.

Yet in the end when fantasy is done,

Back into the box returns my clone,

Erstwhile a clown now gone.

So for a time I'm me again,

Sober and serious, goodness holds the reign,

But still, not far away, beneath the lid,

Is part of me, or all of me,

Of which I'll not be rid,

But which conformity excludes. 2001 (from 'The

plague of 2001 and other poems.')

CHAPTER 7

HOPE AT LAST.

I recall going back to the private hospital for an outpatient appointment with my psychiatrist. He was as usual, unpleasant, and virtually accused me of obtaining my discharge under false pretences. His attitude was singularly unhelpful and I now wish that I had had the strength to stand up to him. When on an earlier occasion and in some desperation, I had phoned him at his other hospital, he had been unpleasant and rude. My trust in this Professor of psychiatry had received a few knocks. When you are ill, you are hypersensitive and extremely vulnerable. Surely this must be known by those treating us. Perhaps such a person is employing some form of shock therapy. Certainly I would never want to see this particular man again. My personal hope now was that hospitals and psychiatrists in them were now in the past. The E.C.T. transformed me. We could now enjoy Christmas and I could look forward to resuming my work.

We decided to spent Christmas itself in the parish, and the Rural Dean, Vicar of St.Augustine's, Bexhill, was so caring and thoughtful. I would let someone else take the Christmas services in my parishes, but I would assist in his church. This went well and was enjoyable. I was so grateful for this priest's care and understanding throughout. Tragically it would not be long before he was to collapse with cancer, and within a short time, he died.

I began to plan my 'come-back'. It was a tradition for the bell ringers at Hooe church to meet on New Year's Eve to ring in the New Year. I suggested that we hold a short watch night service to lead up to the bells. Someone else said that we could have mince pies and mulled wine. I passed on this news to a number of parishioners, and all this was done. It was beautiful, and for me, as the New Year came, I felt new born, emerging at long last from the cruel and other world of depressive, episodic illness.

So I was able to begin my parish ministry properly in Ninfield and Hooe with my Induction in Hooe early in

1991. The church was packed. How good that felt. After all my trials, and knowing what some people's wrong views of mental illness might be, some could have been aloof. But no, the welcome was warm and wonderful and a real vote of confidence. The parishes throughout had been wonderfully patient and understanding, and I had been sent so many messages and cards including from every year in the church primary school, and signed by every pupil. I felt so happy and in a normal non-manic way! The Rural Dean was going to see me from time to time, and of course I would see my own G.P. People, with virtually no exceptions, were warm, supportive and friendly. Life looked decidedly better.

But if E.C.T. had been a turning point, even more effective was to be my G.P.'s next prescription. He said something like this. 'What you have is a chemical disorder of the brain. It is manic-depression, with excessive mood swings.' He went on to say of his prescription,' It isn't an anti-depressant or anything like that. And no-one really knows how it works. What it is is a salt(I think he said). You may not feel any effect for some time, but within a month you'll be feeling a lot better.' The medication ,now taken by so many sufferers, was lithium carbonate, and its effects on my liver and other organs would be monitored every few months by a blood test. Was this, I wondered, what was offered years ago in Croydon when I had opted for an alternative? What a pity I hadn't then chosen lithium. Again I was pleasantly surprised by an almost immediate change. I felt a lot better, not just on the surface, but deep down where all the mental pain had been. My doctor was later to say, ' The good news is that you will never be ill like this again. The bad news is that you will be on lithium for the rest of your life.' The price is worth it!

The result of taking lithium, as other sufferers will know, is that it prevents such big mood swings as I had experienced. It was a kind of topping and tailing of my personality! It provided a kind of safety net for my moods and feelings, suppressing my highs and preventing me from getting too low, but not so much as to take away my natural spontaneity.

I wrote in the Introduction to one of my collections of poems,'…during these years and indeed before, from time to time I suffered from a depressive illness…The condition, I believe ,in retrospect, was both my making and my unmaking. The illness deepened my feelings and perceptions, but may also have affected the shape and contents of my life's work, my career of ministry. But if I had to choose, I think I would embrace creativity and imagination despite the considerable costs.'(Deal Pier and other poems.).

Lithium had not stopped me from composing and preaching sermons, writing, engaging in drama and giving broadcast talks. It is just that the extremes have been tempered, and after being mastered by my mind for so long, I believe myself to be in charge again.

So I continued in my parishes for nearly nine happy years, with only the occasional downs which were not serious and which lasted for no longer that a day or two. I think that people's memories of my grim days largely faded. I think, that together, we achieved a lot, and I made many good friendships. The congregations grew, a new car park was made for Hooe church, and at Ninfield, the possibilities to do the same were explored, all these efforts to accommodate those coming to the churches. When I did decide to retire, some time after reaching sixty, I was given a wonderful send-off. My final sermon was applauded, and it seemed that people were genuinely sorry see me leave.

Writing these words two years after my retirement in 1999,my time proved to be extremely busy, officiating and preaching in different parishes, broadcasting on local radio, acting in the local Players, writing for and directing a church youth drama group. I also published a number of collections of poetry one of which was presented to the Queen Mother in Walmer castle, where My mother and I were received by Her Majesty. I enjoyed as I continue to do, the company of my mother who lives with me. I also enjoy just being in my own home.

And what of the illness? The lithium with the accompanying blood tests continue. and I have the occasional off day or two when I experience a lowering of mood, and sometimes anxiety, but nothing like the months of debilitating depression I have known in the past. The old imaginings sometimes revisit me, and something I may read about or see on television may feed them, e.g. reading about a woman who in 1988 committed a murder she couldn't recall. One possible reason considered was that she had been a forceps delivery. This immediately struck a chord for I too had been delivered in this way, and there is a picture of me as a new born baby with a noticeable lump on my head. There were additional factors in that case I didn't share.

But then it was always a symptom of my illness that anything that could be, was fed in to strengthen my self accusation and self deprecation. In any case, it's just plain silly to think I might have done something like this, for there is no evidence. I have, it would seem, been troubled more by hallucinations that memories of real happenings. By brain may or may not have been affected at birth which may or may not have caused certain errors and shortcomings. But when all is said and done, it is sufficient to be concerned with real mistakes and errors and to try to deal with them, than to be plagued with things that are unlikely and probably imagined. So I have to be more gentle with myself. What I also know is that a 'bruised mind', chemical rather than organic, has been a real and grievous affliction which has overshadowed a major part of my life and ministry.

I am thankful that despite everything that has happened, I have managed to achieve a fair amount except for occasional interruptions. I have never completely given in when my efforts were impossible and the efforts of others were my lifeline. I have tried hard, at times maybe too hard. It would seem that those who have had breakdowns are also often very conscientious. Now, I think that my conscience is more my friend than my tyrant.

Life is sweet again. It is once more a world in which there is plenty of colour but where the colour is restrained and probably more real than the vivid hues of mania. I am so grateful to be happy.

Finally what do I think of this beast, called by some, the 'black dog'? It is suffered by so many, sometimes in a way that's covered up, until it may be too late. These are the silent ones who are in Hell, and cannot bring themselves to tell others of their pain. It is an illness that can go unrecognized by another, for the sufferer may look all right physically and in the early stages. The condition is insidious in its advance, with sleepless nights or an early collapse into sleep and very early waking. It brings acute anxiety, cold or hot sweats, lassitude and a desire to crawl into a private and preferably dark corner. Appetite will go except for brief intervals of gorging, and hope for the future will vanish. Life loses all verve and purpose. There are the additional symptoms of extreme swings of mood.

But all this, with the right help and support can lift. With all my belief in some aspects of the Christian Ministry of Healing, I believe that always the first call should be to a sympathetic and knowledgeable G.P. Anything else that is good and sensible is a bonus.

And what of God in all of this?

At times perhaps I didn't think much of Him. But the Faith of most people receives knocks at times. It is in the perseverance that Faith may be strengthened and shown fresh insights and even grow.. Sometimes I saw events as part of the struggle between good and evil. Certainly at times it felt as if I was under attack by real and palpable evil. But what was precisely going on in my life? I do not really know, save for the awfulness and also an increased awareness and its resulting creativity. Good is always the greater force, and by grace often triumphs. More positively I have learnt a great deal ,though I would never pretend to have any precise medical knowledge. Even psychiatrists seem to be handling an uncertain science. However I really do know what it is to suffer in this way, to have hopes dashed and ambition trampled upon, to be in blackness and to feel alone even when I know I wasn't. And I also know what it is to find recovery and to rediscover the light.

I am not complacent, but I am alive, and life is very good.

My thoughts continue to go out to those who still suffer, in hospital or at home. I feel very much for them for they are heroic souls. What they are going through is horrible. I pray for them. If now you are where I have been, you won't feel like anything positive at present, but on your good days at least, take heart that you can be well again. It may be a very long journey but it is possible for anyone to make it. Then you will join me and many others who have been there, but are now here on the other side of Hell. You will have let the black dog loose.

POSTSCRIPT-UP TO NOW.

My life has continued busy, and on a reasonably even keel. I have continued to assist in a large number of parishes, something I much enjoy, involving as it does, meeting lots of people without the responsibility of being in charge.

I have missed some things, like going to a function where I would be known by everyone, also walking around the villages and being spontaneously greeted, or going into the school to meet children and teachers. In time, even in retirement I am meeting more people spread over a larger area.

In the first of the two villages where I lived in retirement, I joined the drama group. Also requests to officiate soon began to come in from neighbouring parishes. I became a hospital chaplain, working part time for six months. I was asked to join a committee preparing for the Queen's Golden Jubilee celebrations in Dover. I continue my broadcasting by speaking from time to time on B.B.C. Radio Kent. I also continue to write and publish poetry, three books to date. I became Vice Chair of Christians Together in Dover, organising and leading the Good Friday Procession through the town, and also taking 'Songs of Praise' as part of Dover's regatta in 2002 and 2003. I record all this, not to blow my own trumpet but to indicate how far I have come since being seriously ill.

Now, I am in touch with nearly twenty parishes, and in addition to Sunday services, I am sometimes asked to officiate for baptisms, weddings and funerals.

So thanks to lithium, together with the love and support of family and the appreciation of my congregations, my illness is largely held at bay. Hospital and anti-depressants are unnecessary, and sleep is usually natural and good.

Yet occasionally I am reminded of my condition.

If I take on too much at one time, I quickly get exhausted and low.

There was a time recently when I took ten services with eleven preachings including some long distances, all in about a fortnight. I was near despair. At the same time I had to turn down two further requests for funerals, which made me feel guilty.

It was absurd. Anyone would have felt strained!

I do know the symptoms of stress and incipient depression. These are lethargy, exhaustion and irritability, the latter just adding to my feelings of guilt. I also feel sorry for myself and restless at such times.

But the lithium is effective and the crisis period passes, so that for the most part I am stable, productive and not depressed.

Yet there are other reminders.

Whereas I am not particularly manic, I do tend to talk too much and too rapidly at times. I see that glazed look in my listener's eyes. Also I have always tended to entertain the occasional delusion of grandeur, being at times puzzled when my ministry has not been recognized as special by the hierarchy. I relish praise, and feel the sting of disapproval. I hate my mistakes and failings, and can develop anxieties. Visual images as on television make sharp impressions on my senses, so that for a short time after a programme is ended, I still feel part of it, and for a brief time, my home becomes an 'extension' of the set.

So where am I now?

My life is active, happy and mostly illness free. Despite my contact with so many people, there are times when I feel lonely. Because so much of my life has been under the shadow of manic depression, I seem to have lacked the opportunity and the confidence for close friendships or more. This is a greater worry as I get older.

But there are far more positive things about my life, and I believe myself to be very fortunate. The experiences that I have described are a part of my life, therefore of me, a large and very influential part. In some ways now, these bad times seem unreal and very distant. I try not to dwell on them for long or I might again feel threatened.

Yet even the worst times have some positive aspects.

In my ministry to others, my understanding has been deepened and my ability to empathize enhanced. The illness too has helped my powers of imagination, my sensitivity and my creativity. I sometimes wonder if the effects of lithium, in making my mood swings less extreme, have changed my natural personality, causing me to live between a glass ceiling and a safety net. If this is the price to be paid to avoid the profound depths and the absurdly dizzy heights, then so be it. I am happy to pay it.

So all in all, would my life have been better without manic depression? In some obvious ways,ye s, but the illness has admitted me to territory in which the scenery has been more dramatic than the norm, and the insights more vivid, a bit like living in a Walt Disney cartoon. Manic depression has contributed to the person I am, at least as much as all the other parts. We are after all in part the product of all our experiences. In the early days my reaction to illness was perplexity and confusion with not a little resentment. This in time turned to revulsion and shame, bitterness and disappointment. Now I am in calmer waters and I have learned acceptance. Others are now where I was. I hope that they will hang on, so that they too will emerge and know that their present blackness doesn't have to be for ever.   (November 2003.)

p.p.s. In 2005 my mother who had shared my home and had always stood by me, died. The following year, I was taken seriously ill and spent some time in hospital . Yet coming through all this again shows the resilience of the human spirit.

Lightning Source UK Ltd.
Milton Keynes UK
UKHW01f1834170818
327432UK00001B/17/P

9 781847 471024